Light, Dark
the Neuron and the Axon

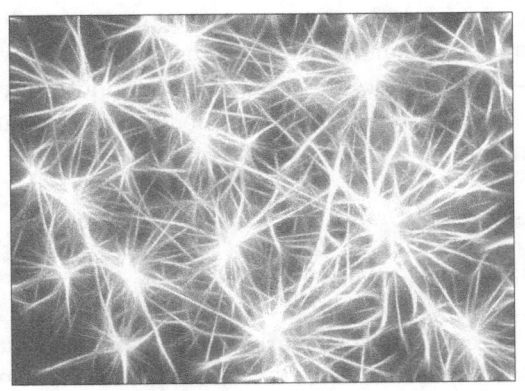

Joseph R. Scogna, Jr.
Kathy M. Scogna

Light, Dark : the Neuron and the Axon
Manuscript by Joseph R. Scogna, Jr., 1984

Copyright © 2014 by Kathy M. Scogna
ALL RIGHTS RESERVED.
No part of this publication may be reproduced, stored in a retrieval system, or transmitted in any form or by any means—digital, electronic, mechanical, photocopying, recording, or otherwise—without the prior permission of the publisher.

Published in the USA by: Life Energy Publications

Cover photo of sparkling, ignited dendrites, PixBay

SAF ® is a registered trademark belonging to Kathy M. Scogna. Its use marks this as the original work of Joseph R. Scogna, Jr.

ISBN-13: 978-1503083080
ISBN-10:150308308X

Light, Dark : the Neuron and the Axon
Includes index, illustrations
1. nervous system 2. DNA 3. energetic healing 4. SAF number system, #12
I. Joseph R. Scogna, Jr. author II. Kathy M. Scogna, author, editor III. Title

Light, Dark
the Neuron and the Axon

Joseph R. Scogna, Jr.
Kathy M. Scogna

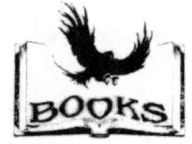

Life Energy Publications
www.LifeEnergyResearch.com

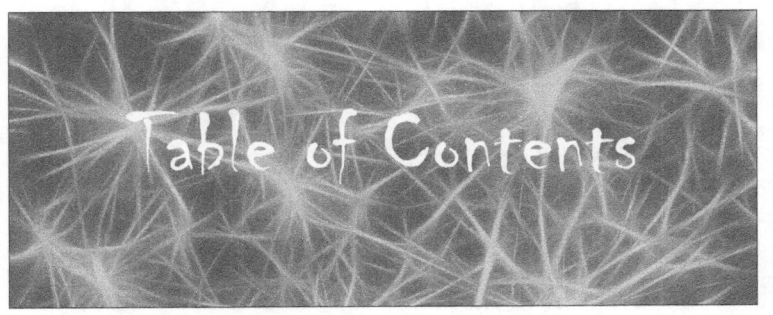

Table of Contents

Introduction by Kathy M. Scogna — 7
Chapter One: The Nerve Cell — 11
   ill. of Nerve cell — 12
   Neuron — 13
   Nucleus of the Neuron — 15
   Nucleolus — 17
   Cytoplasm — 19
   Nissl Bodies — 21
   Chromophil — 23
   Axon Hillock — 25
   Chapter 1. Advanced SAF View — 26
Chapter Two: The Command Center — 27
   ill. of DNA — 28
   DNA — 29
   RNA — 31
   Chapter 2. Advanced SAF View — 32
Chapter Three: Operations — 33
   ill. of Neurons and Nerve Endings — 34
   Peripheral Process — 35
   Central Process — 37
   Dendrites — 41
   ill. of Dendrites — 42
   Axon — 45
   Chapter 3. Advanced SAF View — 47
Chapter Four: Protection of the System — 49

www.LifeEnergyResearch.com

ill. of Protection of the Nervous System — 50
Impulse — 51
Myelin Sheath — 53
Neurilemma — 55
Node of Ranvier — 57
Nucleus of the Schwann Cell — 59
Chapter 4. Advanced SAF View — 62
Neuroglial Cells — 63
Chapter Five: Nerve Cell Personality — 65
ill. of Neurons, Multipolar Neuron — 66
Ions — 67
Unipolar Neuron — 71
ill. of Unipolar Neuron — 72
Bipolar Neuron — 73
ill. of Bipolar Neuron — 74
ill. of Pseudounipolar Neuron — 75
Electric Shock Then and Now — 76
Multipolar Neuron — 77
ill. of Purkinje Nerve Cell — 77
Chapter 5. Advanced SAF View — 79

Epilogue by Kathy M. Scogna — 81
Acknowledgments, References — 84
Credits — 85

Index — 86

Books and Device Mentioned — 90

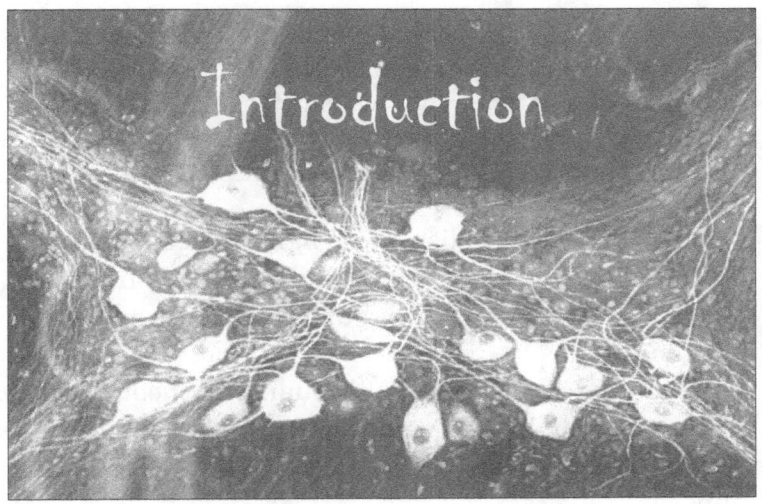

Introduction

*"In the beginning, darkness was over the face of the deep.
And God said, 'Let there be light', and there was light. And God saw that the light was good. And God separated the light from the darkness."*
—Genesis 1:2-4

The illustration above could be an image of stars and galaxies in the night sky, with colliding tails of gas and debris, but instead, the human nerve cells, interconnected by a maze of branching dendrites, are illuminated under a microscope.

Understanding the functioning of the nervous system has been a long process of discovery, which continues even today. But, before man could explore the dark recesses of the human frame and comprehend nerve stimulation, electrical transfers and find what animates the human, he had to first understand light and electricity.

The writers of the Old Testament chose light as their first order of business and described it as a material used by God for the creation of the universe.

Light was that quality that separated the darkness.

In 1690, Dutch mathematician, Christian Huygens, defined what it was that warmed the Earth and lit the skies: light was a form of wave motion, a kind of current that rode the airways from the sun to the Earth.

Sir Isaac Newton dissented: light traveled as a corpuscle (particle), not a wave, and came to Earth from the sun and stars like tiny bubbles drifting on cosmic streams.

Max Planck put forth the quantum theory: basic light is both a particle <u>and</u> a wave, which moves by a magnetic attraction from radiant stars such as our sun.

Quantum comes to us from the Latin, *quantus*, a measurement of *how much*. A quantum is indivisible, the smallest unit, a building block of energy. With quantum physics, we are able to understand the basic underpinnings of matter, the energy and movement of one electron toward another and the transfer of energy between atoms and molecules. It explains the inner workings of matter and energy on the atomic and subatomic levels.

This theory, followed by quantum mechanics, can be applied equally to stars as to atoms, the greatest and the smallest of the cosmos. Eastern philosophies describe this: "As above, so below."

It was quantum mechanics that finally opened the door to explanations of nervous system operations.

Textbooks tells us the human nervous system is the most sophisticated and complex information-processing system in the known universe, which operates at the speed of light as it coordinates, regulates and controls our various organic functions. But, present-day textbooks give us only organic functions, the physical aspects. There is far more to life than mere "organic functions."

In *Light, Dark: the Neuron and the Axon*, life energy researcher, Joseph R. Scogna, Jr. presents a holistic image of the nervous system that cannot be found in any university text.

From an energetic viewpoint, Joe describes the neuron, axon and other components as units that control our life energy, especially the fragmentary dissemination processes of thought, desire, and plans of the genetic mechanism. He assigned SAF® number sequences to these component parts in order that these would meld into his comprehensive Life Energy System and SAF® computer project. The nervous system and the venting sites are intrinsic to his infrared studies. An advanced SAF® view (affected organs and glands) is presented at the end of each chapter.

The nervous system is listed in the SAF® language of organs and glands at #12. This book kindles further comprehension of that #12 system operating in its pure form; knowing this can increase our own awareness and perhaps stimulate others in the future to find ways of correcting nervous system disorders and dysfunctions and leave behind the harmful drugs and electric stimulation (see page 76).

In *Light, Dark: the Neuron and the Axon*, Joe takes us on a futuristic journey into the invisible world within ourselves, to the inner workings of memory, genetics, reception and transmission of stimuli. He lends a voice and personality to the light and dark of the most mysterious, complex circuit known to man, our nervous system.

www.LifeEnergyResearch.com

In many ways, Joe's heart and mind operated in the 25th century with future man.

I invite you on this journey, to explore his exciting work.

—Kathy M. Scogna

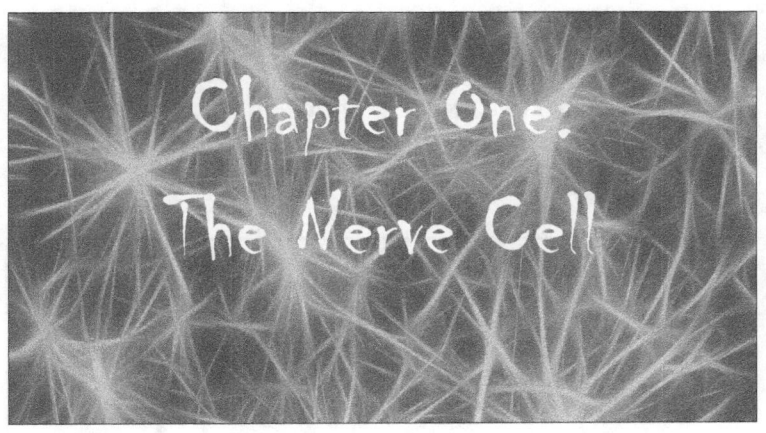

Chapter One: The Nerve Cell

> *"The neuron is the switch mechanism between light and dark in the human structure."*
>
> —Joseph R. Scogna, Jr.

(below) A neuron or nerve cell showing input from branched dendrites, nucleus, nucleolus, cytoplasm, Nissl bodies, axon hillock, axon covered by myelin sheath and neurilemma.

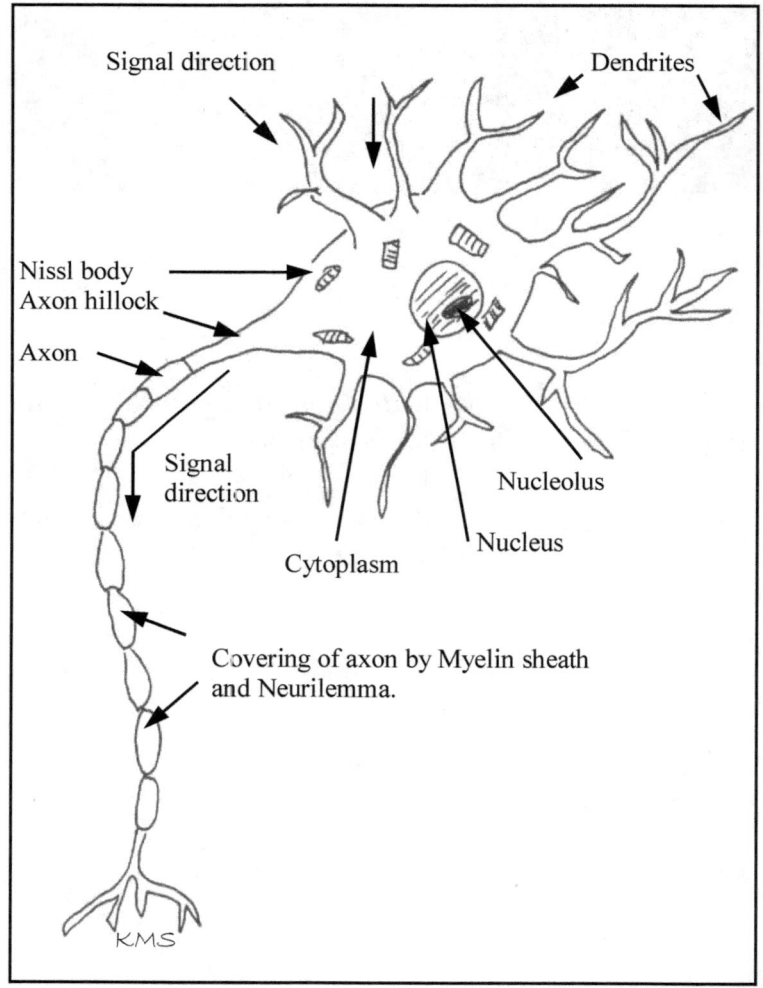

Neuron

The neuron, or nerve cell, is the basic unit of the nervous system, with intrinsic qualities of being. It exists because of the intention of the genetic structure for it to exist, and survives due to the fact that genetic structure and planning mechanism dictate that it survive.* The neuron's purpose is to create a format of acceptance for energy, power, and pressure in the body. The neuron is the switch mechanism between light and dark in the human structure.

The neuron expresses and holds electric pressure and space (lightness and darkness). This electric pressure system and the characteristics of the energies, which it holds onto, can become so intricate and precise that man has yet to discover these infinite variations.

The most sophisticated "computer chip" ever created, the neuron marks off its own space in the body and can calculate faster and with less energy loss than any computing system known to man.

Having the ability to evaluate the results of its efforts, the neuron has correctly built a specific framework of energy, which can analyze and direct activities around it needed for its survival (light) and helps to avoid mortality (dark).

The neuron controls the tempo in the body. Its entire structure is made up of time and specific electrical components, which are fragments of other creations. This means that the system (the nucleus of the neuron and the nucleolus of the neuron) has devel-

---

* for more on the Genetic Planning Mechanism (GPM), see *Junk DNA: Unlocking the Hidden Secrets of Your DNA.*

www.LifeEnergyResearch.com

oped incredibly minute mechanisms for controlling electrochemical processes of the body. These processes are necessary to carry out the dictates of the system.

The neuron is a coordination and equalization unit that controls life energy, especially the fragmentary dissemination processes of thought, desire and plans of the genetic mechanism as well as those plans of the individual himself.

Nucleus of the Neuron

The nucleus is a mechanism that controls the vital fluids inside the neuron, and the quantity of conductant that surges through the neuron structure. (see page 12 for image.)

Except for the nucleolus, the nucleus has a much greater governing control over the neuron than any other structure.

One of the primary functions of the nucleus is the ability to reproduce the entire system; the nucleus can work on specific functions in the body, which help to multiply its significant compensatory energies to refresh and replenish the system. It also has the capability and power of directing and controlling electromagnetic mechanisms, which will help to reproduce regular sustained electric patterns and characteristics that are of benefit to the entire human organism.

A timing mechanism within the nucleus helps to control electric forces, which move about the neuron structure itself. This mechanism depends on pressures (light) and spaces (dark) which shift throughout the sequence of a day. It also has the capabilities of high technological coordination and equalization of pressures and spaces within the system.

Besides all of its other powerful assets, the nucleus has the endowment of analyzation and the ability of creating pressure and space to perform its many multi-faceted functions.

A timing mechanism helps to control electric forces. This mechanism depends on pressures (light) and spaces (dark) which shift throughout the sequence of a day

Nucleolus

The nucleolus starts off its existence out of the spark of experience which is a long-term process handed down by the genetic governors of the body. It has a tremendous ability to create and destroy energies, which are in line with or against the human organism as a whole. (see image page 12)

From the bowels of the nucleolus come messages that cause the system to snap to attention. The energies that are emitted from the nucleolus are much more sophisticated than any coded signals known in the body. The unconscious automatic radio patterns of the nucleolus have not yet been decoded by modern science. These subspace signals have thus far escaped detection by modern scientific instrumentation, because man has elected to observe molecular structures rather than nuclear magnetic resonances. The bowels of the nucleolus also direct actions to be taken for chemical and electrochemical processes occurring on a gross level, visible by normal scientific means. However, the deep-set processes, which are commanded by genetic blueprint, remain hidden in frequency banks which are ultrasonic and of harmonic light and dark in nature.

The nucleolus has very sophisticated powers of evaluation, especially for observing and controlling the results of its desires and intentions. The nucleolus constantly admires its own work, and consistently fights against any interference in the environment that may thwart or disturb its ideals.

The analytical capability of the nucleolus is supreme. It is able to count electrons and subatomic

> *For a body to be able to cope with any environmental upset, it must first be broadcast to the nucleolus in a pattern that is receptive on a nuclear magnetic level.*

particles. It can mathematically dissect and solve any problem in nature, given the right components and the correct electromagnetic and radiational transmission messages from the environment. Since the nucleolus operates on such a small dimension, any gross manifestations of energy which attack its systems may go unnoticed and unprocessed. For a body to be able to cope with any environmental upset, it must first be broadcast to the nucleolus in a pattern that is receptive on a nuclear magnetic level.

The ability of the nucleolus to store power, electric pressures and spaces is cultivated on a very minute and submicroscopic level. The infinitesimally small energies that are used by this system are almost incomprehensible, but nonetheless are the precursors for many of the electromagnetic and electrochemical structures of the system.

The nucleolus is a sophisticated mechanism of coordination and tempo. The timing mechanisms of this minute part of the neuron are beyond measure at this point in time. The only mechanisms that are more accurate than the nucleolus are those that are concocted by the mind and the spirit themselves.

Cytoplasm

Cytoplasm is the circulating energy around the nerve cell. It is the aqueous material that permits movement and creation of energy within the boundaries of the cell walls and can be seen in the image on page 12.

Cytoplasm has the ability on its own to direct and control activities that happen on the playing field. It has its own resistance, which can be measured in pico-ohms (this is a trillionth of an ohm—written 1×10^{-12}). There are also forces within the cytoplasm that can be measured in femto-ohms and atto-ohms resistance, which are quadrillionths (1×10^{-15}) of an ohm and quintillionths (1×10^{-18}) of an ohm, respectively. The latter of the two is perhaps the boundary of cytoplasm. This however, does not thwart the other mechanisms of the cell, especially the nucleolus, from going beyond this measurement.

The cytoplasm has the ability to carry on metabolism of energies around the cell; it harbors energies that can coordinate and direct the activities of digestion, detoxification and purification of the cell substances.

The cytoplasm also supplies the special waters and fluids needed for conductivity of energies from the cortex of the nerve cell to the nucleus and the nucleolus.

Energies of the cytoplasm eventually send signals by means of nucleic and ribonucleic acids to coordinate energies as the building blocks of proteins, necessary for the creation of bones and muscles. The cytoplasm of the nerve cell (neuron) is more intrinsi-

> *Energies of the cytoplasm eventually send signals by means of nucleic and ribonucleic acids to coordinate energies as the building blocks of proteins, necessary for the creation of bones and muscles.*

cally connected with the dissemination of control processes in the body, which help to keep the system neurologically fit so it can subsist in this environment.

Cytoplasm is a substance that demarcates and cordons off other energies from it. Each neuron, although extremely similar to other neurons, has its own specialty and individuality. Energies from within the nucleolus push outward to form the perimeter of the neuron. The energies therein then seek to establish themselves as a unique and characteristic force.

Nissl Bodies

The Nissl bodies, or Nissl substance, were named after Franz Nissl, who discovered these transmitters of data within the cell membrane. Also called *tigroid* due to their tiger-like stripes, they are intimately connected with protein synthesis and metabolism, and are premiere transmitters of data to the system. The energies directed from these Nissl bodies help coordinate the activities and functions of the neuron itself.

These substances are composed of an endoplasmic network (reticulum) found within the cytoplasm of the neural cell, see illustration on page 12.

The Nissl bodies also contain energies that can hold onto and deal with foreign energies in the nervous structure. They possess their own self-protective mechanisms to coordinate forces in the neuron having lysosomal activity; these lysosomes (enzymes) are able to break down poisons and detoxify the system.

In view of the cardinal mechanism of the Nissl body, the structure develops a keen sense of awareness when contending with energies that do not belong within its perimeters. The Nissl body has the power to send signals of rejection to all such energies.

The structure of the Nissl body adds a sense of high quality to the neuron. It acts as a transmitter-radio station that upgrades the relay of information in the system. It is like a star librarian or grand educator.

The metabolic processes of the Nissl body also contain many secrets, which were once the prizes of alchemists. The transmutational capabilities of the Nissl bodies are very powerful; they are capable of

> *The Nissl bodies contain energies that can hold onto and deal with foreign energies. This is a self-protective mechanism to coordinate forces in the neuron having lysosomal activity (enzymes) that are able to break down poisons and detoxify the system.*

translating one element into another. The relative structure of the Nissl body (a cylindrical shape) acts very much like the thalamus of the midbrain; it is a coordinator and translator of light and dark impulses.

Finally, the Nissl body has the sense and capability of digesting energies, especially proteins, molecules, atoms, and electrons, and translating them into substances that are more closely coordinated with the overall plans, dreams, and desires of the system as a whole.

Chromophil

The chromophil is a neurosecretory cell that is easily stained and is found throughout the body. It is one of two types of cells in the pituitary gland. It releases hormones from the pituitary as well as the hypothalamus, thyroid, parathyroid and the pancreas.

The word chromophil means, *"love for color."* The chromophil has a prismatic effect and is part of the neuron structure itself. The nervous system has an entourage of energies that contribute to its overall splendor of operation, and the chromophil is the mechanism transmitting these messages in more colorful terms. (Light = all color; dark = no color).

Chromophils have digestive capabilities similar to the Nissl bodies. The probable reason for this is that the chromophil is actually a type of Nissl body. It also possesses the ability to detoxify the system.

Conditions of action and metabolization are part and parcel of the chromophilic behavior. This mechanism changes color and energy into metabolites on a nervous cellular basis.

The qualities of the fluids around the nerve cell (the neuron) are tempered by the chromophil, which has the capabilities of transmutating energies around the cells to suit itself.

With the powers of direction and coordination, the electromagnetic influence of the chromophil draws proteins and other cellular particles into its network and retranslates them into a signal that can be delivered to another nerve cell or ganglion. The pyramidal structure of the nervous system is constructed so as to preclude any haphazard activity on

> *Chromophil means "love for color." It has a prismatic effect and is part of the neuron structure.*
>
> *The nervous system has an entourage of energies that contribute to its overall splendor of operation, and the chromophil is the mechanism transmitting these messages in more colorful terms. (Light = all color; dark = no color).*

the part of chromophils. In other words, there is a precise chain of command causing the energies to systematically issue directives and orders to the higher structures of the body.

Axon Hillock

An axon hillock is an eminence or projection coming out of the neuron so that the axon itself can extend from it. It is like a cylindrical cuff that allows the axon to emit from the neuron. It is likely that the Nissl bodies themselves are potential axon hillocks or energies, which may eventually proliferate and transform the unipolar or bipolar neuron into the multipolar mechanism. If the Nissl bodies move toward the perimeters of the neuron, they could actually make axon hillocks, which could then in turn create projections from the axons to produce more service area of the cell.

The axon cylinder, or axon hillock, has powers of transmutation. Like many of the structures within the nerve cell, light and dark radiation is degraded and upgraded into specific structures which are compatible with the overall system.

The axon hillock also has capabilities of detoxification and containment. Apparently, the entire system has a particular resistance running across its magnetic trails. The power and energy within the nervous system is constantly being thwarted by the overall resistance and the tempered conductance of the system. The axon hillock itself has a specific amount of resistance to offer; however, in electrical terms it is measured in pico ohms (trillionths of an ohm).

The specific materials that nourish the axon hillock are specialized in that they are directed to carry on processes of metabolization and transmutation of energies, the primary mechanism of operation for the system.

The power and energy within the nervous system is constantly being thwarted by the overall resistance and the tempered conductance of the system. The axon hillock has a specific amount of resistance to offer; however, in normal terms it is measured in pico ohms (trillionths of an ohm).

The action and metabolization of energies are part of the electrical transfer process from one neuron to the other and must be carefully guarded by the axon hillock. This cuff is a specialized filter that prevents the straying of any energies traveling from one neuron to another neuron.

The control of electromagnetic energies, especially current measured in trillionths of amperes and specific energy transfer processes, are too incomprehensible to measure at present.

The tempo of energy passing from the neuron through the axon can be directly controlled by the axon hillock. The energies therein have a specific capability of disallowing pressures that are too great or too deficient from escaping the neuron itself.

Chapter 1.—Advanced SAF® View

The organs and glands primarily affected are: pituitary (5 and 21), brain (12), mind (14), liver (6), thyroid (10) endocrine system (17/18), adrenals (13), and colon (3).

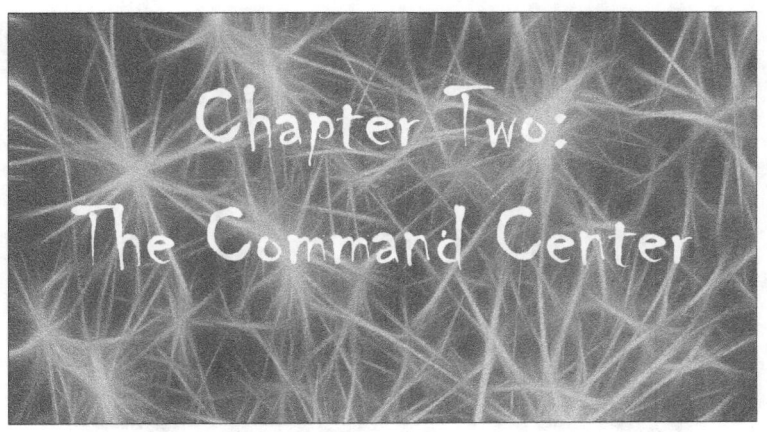

Chapter Two: The Command Center

> *"Operating under the strict rules of time, tempo, and procedure, the RNA is a synchronized mechanism controlling, harboring and relaying electricity."*
>
> —Joseph R. Scogna, Jr.

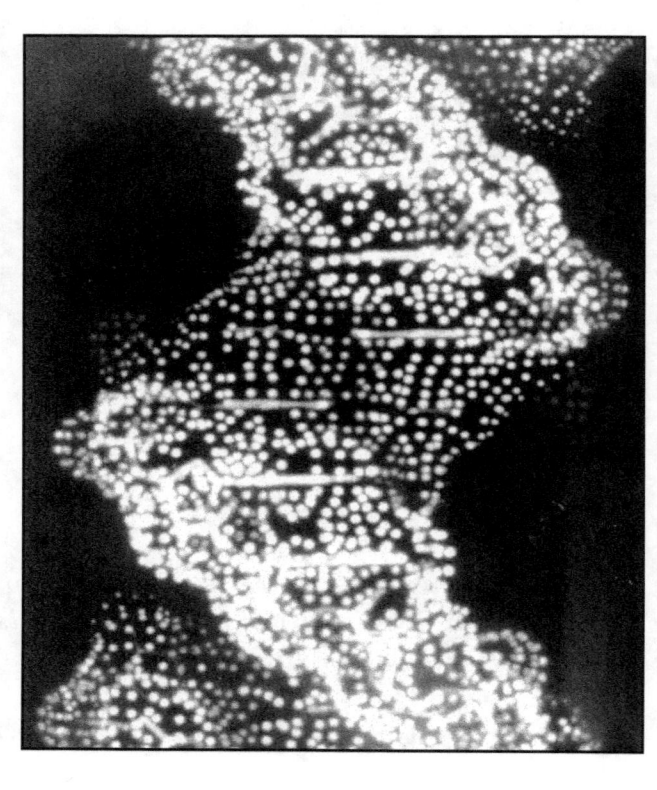

Image of DNA

To a chemist, DNA is a very rigid study, which adheres to the rules and laws of physical chemistry and visible lab work.

The DNA addressed with SAF® is accessible through very intense mental and spiritual conditioning. This is accomplished with our own personal SAF chain work following the laws of electricity and physics.

DNA (deoxyribonucleic acid)

Perhaps the DNA is the most intrinsic part of the cellular structure. The genetic molecular code for each cell is entrusted to this mechanism. It is the selective unit necessary for the competent and proficient running of the overall human system.

The DNA has endowed itself with the abilities of evaluation, especially for any effects created by it or the environment on the organism. The DNA must be able to systematically observe and analyze the activities of all other energy forces surrounding the molecule, especially from one cell to another.

The DNA analyzation capabilities are specific in their ability to cordon off various spaces of operation. This may be one of its most powerful activities. The DNA establishes its location of operation via its inherited genetic plan.

The specific fluids that surround the DNA are in precise quantities, which can be translated by a crystalline mirror-like structure, like a laser beam, throughout the entire system. Thus the passages of processes throughout the entire system, whether they be electrical, electrochemical, or purely chemical, can follow a precise mirrored blueprint.

The actions of the DNA and RNA are necessary to put the whole system into operation.

The coordinating and equalizing efforts of the DNA and RNA are such that they create energy bias producing a homeostasis of survival or existence. The DNA and RNA combination of elements causes a specific and relative distinction between what is truly inert and actually kinetic as far as energy goes. In other words, the DNA and RNA structure stabilizes, controls, and activates energy in the system.

What is in our DNA? Everything we have needed to survive for these past millennia. From the hardwired fabric of the universe since the beginning of time, approximately 4 billion years ago, including what has occurred on and in the Earth, to our individual inheritances and lifetime events, all is stored in our DNA. *

Detoxification and energy awareness are necessary for understanding and accessing the DNA-RNA programs. The introduction of hormones and other concentrated drug materials cause the DNA-RNA to react and write new script into its transmitting banks to try to counteract the onslaught of extraneous iatrogenic poisons. There is enough coming from the environment itself without adding to the situation.

---

* For a complete rundown of the 16 Steps of the Z Process (what is hardwired in to the DNA) to the 128 sensory channels of perception (what is accessible to us), read *Junk DNA: Unlocking the Hidden Secrets of Your DNA*.

RNA (ribonucleic acid)

The RNA is the message center and coordinator of protein in the system, having the capability of evaluating its own handiwork. It looks at the results of its creations and sends information back to the DNA for further instructions.

RNA, which is an entity in itself, has the ability to code, regulate, decode and to reject plans, ideas, and instigation from the DNA. It can judge and discern whether or not a plan will be good for the host, the life energy body; however, most of its efforts are directed towards automatically carrying out commands of the DNA.

Storing and hoarding power is another capability of RNA. Many times when an individual is hypoglycemic or losing energy, it is due to the fact that the RNA is actually collecting and controlling energies in the system to facilitate one big corrective measure or specific genetic change.

The RNA is extremely receptive to information. It must be a "good listener" in order to have the ability of re-describing, interpreting and transmitting information to other less sophisticated protein structures.

With the capabilities of defense, the RNA can protect the DNA against invasions and toxic incursions from the outside, which seek to alter or mutate its structures.

Operating under strict rules of time, tempo, and procedure, the RNA is a synchronized mechanism controlling, harboring, and relaying electricity.

Note: While a chemist views DNA from a rigid and often purely physical stance, the DNA and RNA addressed with SAF® processing is accessible to us through very intense mental and spiritual conditioning. This is personal work; not found under a microscope. There is much to uncover and relearn how to use.

Chapter 2.—Advanced SAF® View

The organs and glands primarily affected are: hypothalamus and the senses (15) and the spleen (23).

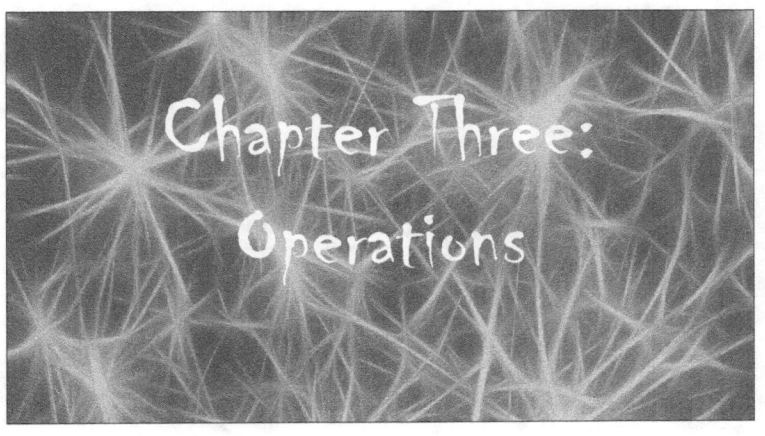

Chapter Three: Operations

> "The body is a hologram. It is a three dimensional image of colored light and non-colored darknesses (invisible), which depend on the crystalline structures of nerve cells and 800 trillion other cells."
>
> —Joseph R. Scogna, Jr.

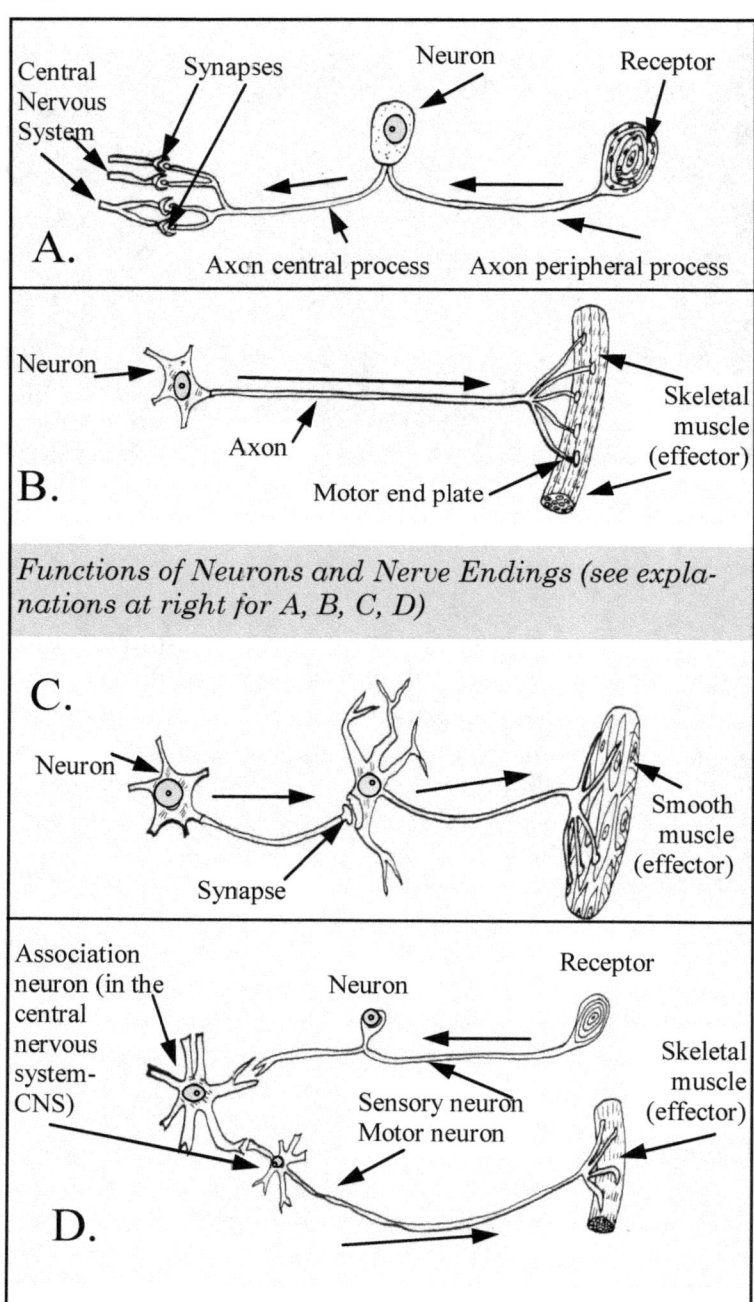

Functions of Neurons and Nerve Endings (see explanations at right for A, B, C, D)

Peripheral Process

The peripheral processes of the neuron are the axons and dendrites outside the cell body. These are the structures that work in conjunction with the cell body to allow one neuron to communicate with another, see A. on chart page 34.

A peripheral process primarily filters transmissions and receptions from one cell to the other in a way similar to human communication on a grand scale. The listener chooses what he wants to hear. The activities around the cell are set up in periods of harmonic motion, which permit certain transmissions to reach the cell body and others to pass right through it. The filtering process of the cell body is capable of discerning the differences and similarities of light and dark, wavelength and frequency, as well as the modulation of these from one cell body to the next. In this way, the cell can selectively communicate with other nerve cells. The cell body can respond, react or give commands to other nerve cells or any other kind of cell in the body by utilizing this filtration process.

(left) Functions of Neurons and Nerve Endings.
A. *Sensory Neuron (afferent—information from receptor to neuron to synapse to central nervous system-CNS).*
B. *Somatic motor neuron (efferent—from neuron to skeletal muscle).*
C. *Autonomic motor neuron (efferent—from neuron to synapse to smooth muscle)*
D. *Association neuron in the central nervous system-CNS (from receptor to neuron through CNS association neurons to skeletal muscle).*

The synchronization of activity around the neuron allows it to sustain operations. Without this filtration system, the operations of the nerve cell would cease to function. The peripheral processes help to circulate energies in and out of the cell body. All motion and movement can be controlled by these mechanisms.

The change of energies, that is, the actual degradation and reintegration of particles and energies to and from the cell body, can be controlled by the peripheral processes. This means that the peripheral processes act like a sophisticated secretary for a high level executive. The secretary is able to screen mail and visitors which may annoy or disrupt the functions of the executive. The peripheral processes (the dendrites and axons) have the ability to coordinate functions as well as to edit and delete certain communications that may not be savory for the cell body itself.

Being physical entities as well as electrical entities, the peripheral processes can substantially mark off areas around the cell and around other nerve cells to broadcast a pattern to other entities in the body that these pressures and spaces belong to this particular cell. This means that the peripheral processes can reject the encroachment of other cellular entities and therefore mark off a territory for operation.

The movement of the cell in time and space is necessarily tempered by the poles outside the neuron. These poles (the peripheral processes) have the ability to hold onto and move energies, which are part of the physical and electrical makeup of the nerve cell. This means that the peripheral processes can choose whether or not to allow the nerve cell to exist.

Central Process

The central process is the main body of the nerve cell (see A page 34).

Actions and activities of the electronic nerve cell include its ability to transmutate, reserve, and waste energy. The nerve cell enjoys its endowment with one particular, all-encompassing power on a micro scale: that is, to be able to change one color (light and dark) into another or to change chemical and electrical processes, remolding energies to suit its fancy.

The action of transmutation bestows the central processes with the ability to run the entire mechanism. This means that much of the selective body, or the mass of unified cells, depends primarily on the ability of one cell to transmit a sophisticated message to another cell. The cells that create the most workable survival plans are the central control cells. Even after a survival plan is concocted, however, the central process must then broadcast and disseminate it to the other nerve cells. The neurons transmitting from axons to the dendrites of other neurons in this way are able to share information on a unilateral basis. This means that the neurons that are on a par operating level can share information with each other.

The sharing of information causes the mechanism to need an extremely sophisticated communication exchange; processes that are developed cannot be inhibited by normal communication channels. There must be a highly technical methodology of communication between nerve cells that is harmonic and direct. The communication by protein mechanisms floating through the blood stream is too slow for this purpose. Therefore, the mechanism of the central process has developed a sophisticated laser-like approach to communication. Energies can be transmitted simultaneously to every cell in the body at the speed of light, 186,000 miles per second, by using harmonic light and dark at various frequency ranges. Some of the ranges that are used are the electric, microwave, radio, infrared, and ultraviolet bands. In more sophisticated processes, the x-ray, gamma, and cosmic bands are also used. Much of the message that is broadcast to other cells has to do with the correction and substantiation of activities which occur in a visible light spectrum, i.e. color (light) and absence of color (dark).

The central process, after gaining its ability to communicate, is much more able to analyze and judge dimensions in the body. This is an extremely important ability, for the nervous system must be able to get a relative idea as to how much index, current, and resistance is needed to establish homeostasis of color in the body.

To create the proper holographic picture of an individual, the nervous system, and especially those more complicated multi-polarity neurons are needed to direct electrical energy in harmonic ways to contain the process of holography. The body itself is a hologram. It is a three-dimensional image of colored light and non-colored darknesses (invisible) which depends on the crystalline structures of nerve cells and the 800 trillion other cells that receive and transmit information concerning the configuration of the body.

The holographic view of the body, which is part and parcel of the activities of the central process of the nerve cell, must be able to courageously observe electric pressures (voltages). The capacity of each nerve cell must be in tune with the overall genetic program dictating how an individual's body will look.

The consistent and final coordination and equalization of the aforementioned processes must be extremely precise. Some of the tolerances that are necessary to perform these miraculous feats of energy are beyond normal, average understanding. This does not mean, however, that the human being cannot learn to control these processes by utilizing mechanisms and tools that are on an equal dimensional level to the central process. Specific to this idea are the infrared sensors used in the SAF® method to detect areas of heat, which translates into heated or stressed organ and gland systems. (see IR 200 device on page 90.)

Peripheral and Central Processes
When the impulse is moving IN this is a peripheral process. When the impulse is moving OUT, this signifies the central process.
Afferent and Efferent
When the impulse is moving toward the central nervous system (CNS), this is afferent. When the impulse is moving away from the CNS, it is efferent

Dendrites

The dendrite is the receptor of the nerve cell. It is the mechanism that uses energy from the nerve cell to receive information from other nerve cells and other input from the body and the environment surrounding the body.

The dendrite has abilities of judging results; it must evaluate any energy that flows toward it. The minute terminals that are used as receptors for the dendrite cause a synaptic connection. This means that the dendrite has capabilities permitting it to sensor information coming into the central process of the cell body. In many ways, the dendrite can also act as a circuit breaker. If the incoming information is of too fast or too random a particle flow, the dendrite has the ability to disallow its entrance into the nerve cell or neuron.

The activity of the dendrite and its ability to evaluate and control the entrance of information into the cell body allows its own existence. Its control of resistance to electrical flow is a realizable energy force, which creates a certain standard of security for each nerve cell. The behavior of the cell itself depends greatly upon the dendrite, since it controls many of the acceptance and rejection processes around the cell.

The metabolization of energies, that is, specifically the breakdown and buildup of particles for digestion of the nerve cell, may begin in the dendrite. All action taken toward the nerve cell itself must be screened or coordinated by the dendrite.

The tree-like structure of the dendrite gives it the ability to stretch out its tendrils and connect with axons. The axons flowing out from another cell body are able to push energy away from other nerve cells toward receptive neurons. The dendrite is then able to circulate the information going from one nerve cell to the other. It is up to the nerve cell to train the dendrite directly so that policies of acceptance and rejectance are consistent with the rest of the organism.

The dendrite has a very accurate experience track. Since energy from one cell to the other is flowing directly through it, dendrites have the ability to record experiences of energy passing from one nerve cell to the other. In this way, the dendrite behaves much like a recording machine, which can accurately access and read back automatically, any information

(below) The tree-like dendrite is the receptor for the nerve cell. It receives information from other nerve cells, evaluates it and controls the entrance of information into the neuron cell body.

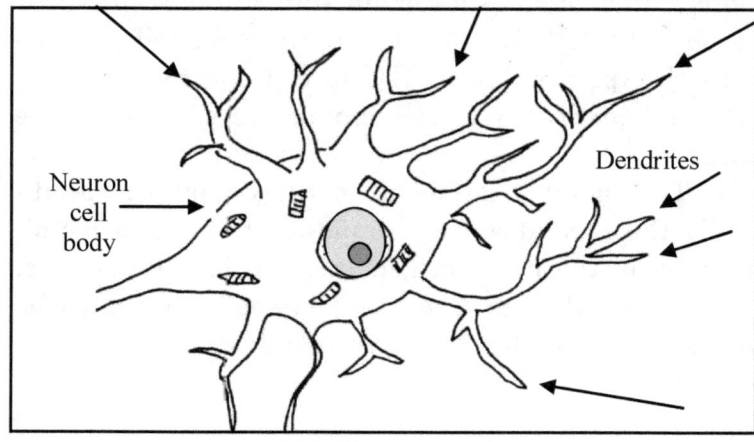

> *Dendrites have the ability to record experiences of energy passing from one nerve cell to the other. In this way, the dendrite behaves much like a recording machine, which can accurately access and read back automatically, any information passing through it. This makes the dendrite one of the most sophisticated devices in the body.*

passing through it. This makes the dendrite one of the most sophisticated devices in the body.

Because the dendrite is connected with programs and processes allowing it to control time in the body, it often becomes backed up with information processing and causes the individual to experience the phenomenon of time passing too slowly. This is due to a high-pressure system building up around the dendrite atmosphere. As energies are processed through the dendrite and finally the high-pressure systems are relieved, the individual may begin to experience a sense that time is passing normally or in some cases may be passing very quickly.

The passage of time as a perception from one person to another relies on the amount of pressure or electric pressure (voltages) which must be changed.

Higher voltages than normally experienced, often create the illusion of time moving too slowly.

Lower voltages, however, create a sense that time is moving very quickly.

The difference between these two phenomena depends greatly on how fast the dendrite can process electrical information from one nerve cell to the other.

Axon

The axon is a mechanism that draws a straight line out from the central nerve cell process. By definition, the axon is a positive structure. Any energy moving out away from another body is considered positive (light); any energy moving in toward a body is considered negative (dark). The synchronized activity of the axon is endowed by the central nerve processes (neurons, nucleolus and nucleus), that are especially interested in transmitting specific positive messages from one cell to the other. Because the cell's overall purpose is continued immortality and constant survival, the messages sent from one cell to the other are often bits of information helping the overall system to become much more harmonic. A primary axiom of energy states that systems will become more harmonic in order to survive in this universe, and less harmonic or disharmonic when succumbing. If one is interested in winning, he must first organize himself and become greatly synchronized with the environment. In the same sense, if one is losing and not attaining the goals that he wishes, then he is most certainly disharmonic in a specific area.

The axon is also part of the nerve cell's armaments. Due to the fact that the nerve cell possesses such positive electrical powers (voltages), it regards these as gold, money or energy that is prized. Since it must protect itself, the axon can act like a weapon.

> *A primary axiom of energy states that systems will become more harmonic in order to survive in this universe, and less harmonic or disharmonic when succumbing.*

> *The axon transmits information and records this information in a positive sense; it is a recording of transmissions.*

The electrical charge sent as a communication message, may be transmutated or degraded to another type of piercing attack mechanism that may sting an invading force or intruder.

The circulation and movement of energy from one cell body to the next is the bailiwick of the axon. After the system is fully protected against any invaders, the axon is much more capable and relaxed about sending transmissions to and from other cell bodies. This department of the axon is an area segmented from its normal duties of protection. In a sense, the axon is able to wear many different hats to accomplish the specific goal of translating and transmitting information from one cell body to the other.

The analyzation of activities and the discernment of time and space are extremely important to the axon, for it is part of the energy expenditure of the cell body needed to communicate with another cell body. In other words, the axon is able to do a "cost benefit study" on its ability to move from one cell body to the next and transmit its load of information concerning the survival plans of the neuron from whence it came.

Like the dendrite, the axon has tremendous capabilities of recording. Unlike the dendrite, the axon transmits information and records this information in a positive sense; it is a recording of transmissions rather than a recording of receptions, as in the case of the dendrite.

The equalization process that is part of the axon's nature is necessary to coordinate the activities of communication messages sent from one cell body to the next. This means that the axon is able to censor information transmitted from the nerve cell that may be detrimental to the receiving nerve cell.

Chapter 3.—Advanced SAF® View

The organs and glands primarily affected are: heart (2) thyroid (10, parathyroid (22), veins and arteries (11), and endocrine system (17/18).

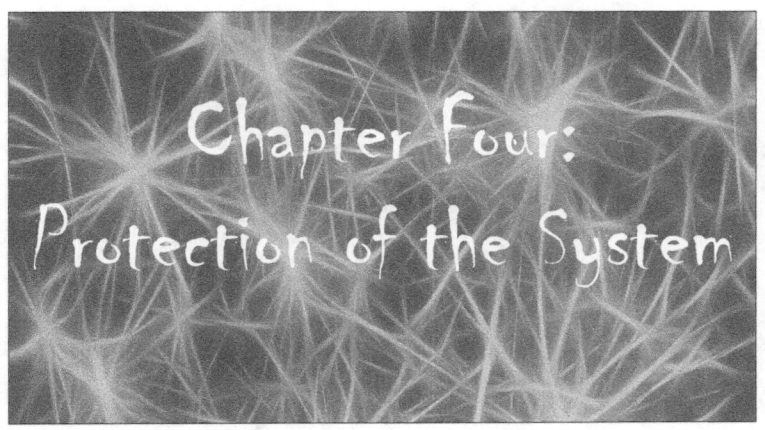

Chapter Four: Protection of the System

> *"The ability to capture, hold and move energies from one area to the other by being resistive to electric charge is part of the directive energy which steers the highly charged atoms down the conduit of the axon."*
>
> -Joseph R. Scogna, Jr.

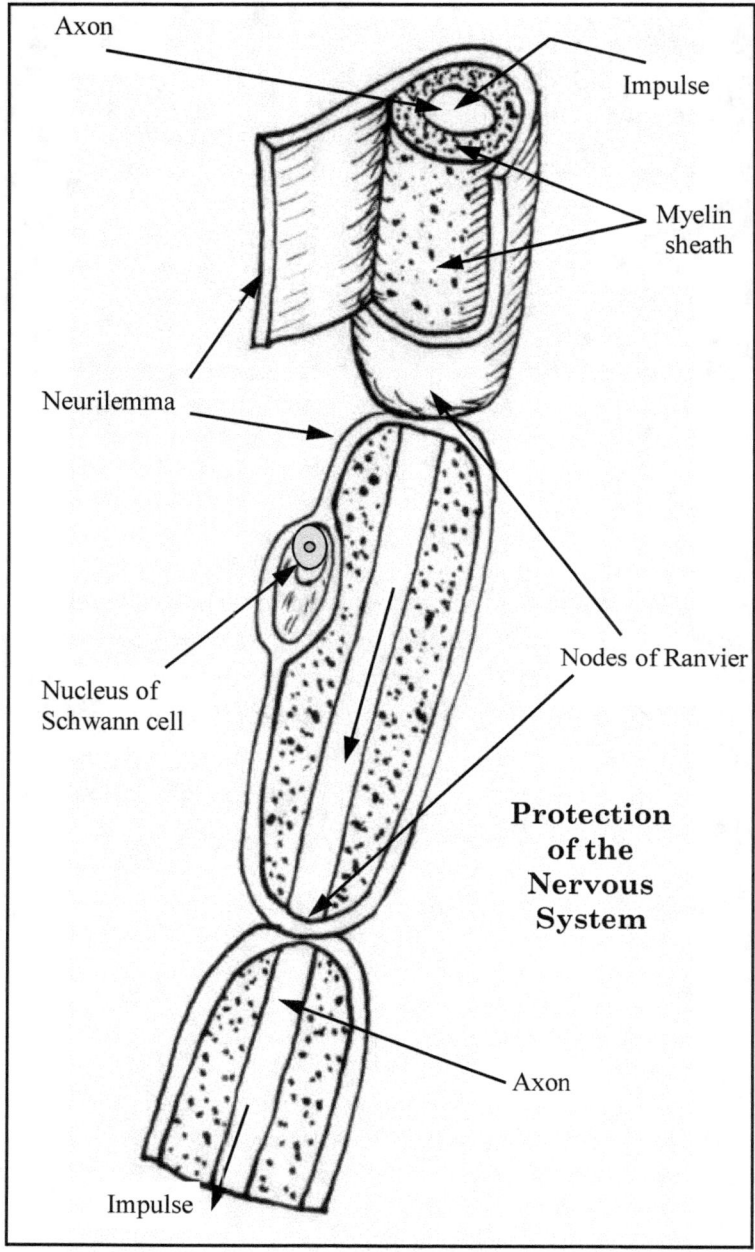

Protection of the Nervous System

Impulse

An impulse is a communications signal from one nerve cell to another. Nerve impulses, also called spikes or action potentials, consist of electrically-charged atoms or ions, the preparation of which involves the arrangement of electrons (subatomic particles).

Impulse acceptance is an extremely important feature of the nerve cell mechanism that delivers it. The cellular membranes, which fire impulses along axons to dendrites, must be able to accept charges. This acceptance of charge can be measured along the axon and dendrite and requires the proper release of sodium ions to open the gateway. Following the sent message or impulse, potassium channels open and allow a return to a resting state. In this way, the impulse can only move in one direction.

The rejection of charge must be in opposition to the impulse acceptance. In normal electrical jargon, this would be the current (impulse) versus the resistance (measured in ohms).

The nerve cell or central process of the nerve cell governs the location and quality of the impulse; it is a message that is broadcast in an effort to create harmony. Breakdown of this message and toxification or corruption of the encoded inscription of electrically charged atoms causes a disharmony of energy within the body.

(left) Protection of the nervous system: the myelin sheath and neurilemma surround the axon, which carries the impulse, to insulate and protect it from outside influence and excess electric charge.

> *The nerve cell or central process of the nerve cell governs the location and quality of the impulse; it is a message that is broadcast in an effort to create harmony. Breakdown of this message and toxification or corruption of the encoded inscription of electrically charged atoms causes a disharmony of energy within the body.*

The outward push of the impulse helps to establish the whereabouts of the cell. Evaluation of its own results is another capability of the impulse. Even though the energy must be directed and coerced to perform its specific functions, the electrical impulse fired from nerve cells is endowed with a sophisticated sensor mechanism, similar to an infrared heat-seeking missile. It is able to evaluate the results of its energies on a very primitive and limited scale.

Myelin Sheath

The myelin sheath is composed of concentric layers, seen as a protective coating around the axon on page 50. It is an insulator, working the same way rubber does around the conducting part of an electrical wire. It has the capability of demarcating energies in order to keep electrical impulses and charges following along the intended pathways of the axon. With all electrical systems, the resistance and component parts of the energies surrounding the transmission diffuse the power and capabilities of that transmission. Myelin energies are an insulating fat membrane preventing the transmutation or escape of energy outside of its barriers.

The exchange between the myelin sheath and the conducting part of the axon (composed of highly conductive materials arranged in a chain link fashion) takes place intimately. The vaporization of electric gases between the conducting part of the axon and the myelin sheath allow both to co-exist, for the myelin sheath is an entity that repulses electric charge. Therefore, there must be a meeting ground or an area that is compatible for both, permitting the myelin sheath to provide its protection for the conducting area of the axon.

With the capability of mending and repairing itself, the myelin sheath attracts energies from the body to reproduce its structural configuration. The myelin compound is a fat-like substance consisting of cholesterol, certain cerebrosides (fatty substances found in brain tissue) and phospholipids. Myelin also includes presence of fatty acids. Its cellular makeup

> *The myelin sheath is endowed with capabilities of rejecting energies that are in high motion.*
> *The protection capability of myelin is only as good as the integrity of the overall autoimmune protective system itself.*

is chemically composed of energies that resist water and electric pressure.

The myelin sheath is endowed with capabilities of rejecting energies that are in high motion. Electrochemical impulses, highly charged atoms, and even electrons bounce off its structure, traveling down the conduit of the axon to send specific messages from one cell to another.

The ability to capture, hold and move energies from one area to the other by being resistive to electric charge is part of the directive energy that steers the highly charged, excited atoms down the conduit of the axon.

Most auspiciously, the myelin sheath establishes a skirmish line that disallows any stray energies from either moving in toward and interfering with the messages from the axon, or moving out of the area, dispersing them. The protection capability of myelin, however, is only as good as the integrity of the overall autoimmune protective system itself.

In the case of an autoimmune demyelinating disease, such as multiple sclerosis, there is extensive loss of the protecting myelin. As mentioned, the myelin has the capability of mending and repairing itself in some cases. When remyelination occurs, partial or complete recovery periods follow.

Neurilemma

The neurilemma is a husk-like sinew or a thin membranous sheath surrounding nerve fibers, as seen on the illustration on page 50. It plays a substantial role in the regeneration of peripheral nerves.

The circulatory actions of electrostatic and dynamic charges are controlled by neurilemma as part of the axon covering that works with myelin.

The neurilemma is a protective mechanism thwarting the interference of axon transmissions. It has high capabilities of regenerating itself.

The neurilemma has the ability to hold and even correct charges, which may be angling off into other directions. In many cases, the neurilemma behaves similarly to the myelin sheath.

However, the neurilemma is much more able to filter particular types to charge particles, allowing some energy through, while the myelin is much more stubborn about demarcating areas of the axon.

With the capability of recording experiences of energy passing through it, the memory of the neurilemma can be played back and re-experienced. Myelin is inferior to the neurilemma in this aspect.

The demarcation abilities of neurilemma are as precise as myelin, pushing away energies which are not of its own kind. The magnetic attractive ability of myelin is much greater than neurilemma; however, both can acquire similar molecular materials for their own regeneration.

> *The neurilemma is capable of recording experiences of energy passing through it; these memories can be played back and be re-experienced.*

Node of Ranvier

Viewing the image on page 50, the node of Ranvier is seen as a junction box between one axon section with Schwann cell to another axon section with Schwann cell. The node of Ranvier is the coupling between them. It was named for anatomist Louis-Antoine Ranvier who discovered the nodes and gaps in 1854.

The node of Ranvier is a very specific energy device that actually envelops and digests one message then recapitulates it for transmission to the next Schwann cell. Often the activity of this digestion and reintegration permits the Schwann cell to contain an entire message without disturbing the information one iota. This is the idea or concept of teleportation. There is some loss of charge doing this, however, to transmit information across space in such an extremely rapid and powerful way, the construction of the nodes of Ranvier are most delicate and sophisticated.

Energies that are exchanged from one cell to another are in the form of charged atomic gas particles. In this way, the vaporization process from one exchange to the next is not hampered by resistance of any electron processes within metals or other types of solid objects that may inhibit the communication of the message from one source to the next.

The nodes of Ranvier are extremely acceptant. In fact, the acceptance level of the node is 100% in a healthy, functioning axon. The Schwann cells are designated to carry coded messages in the form of charged atoms and to send them down the axon with the correct speed and potential dictated from the central process of the nerve structure.

Having the incredible capability of attracting similars and reproducing them, the nodes of Ranvier can make exact copies of messages that are sent from one energy to the next. In many ways, the structure itself is like a mirrored prism; reflections of light are bounced angularly through the axon structure so that this highly charged atomic gas chamber can harmonize the energies within the axon into a laser-like system. Therefore, the harmonic message received on the other end of the transmission is an exact duplicate of the message that was sent.

Filtration and refusal are abilities of the node of Ranvier utilized to prevent any interference from hampering transmission of encoded messages through its systems. It also allows the specific energies in the system that are inscribed with messages to move from one neuron to the other. In a sense, the node of Ranvier is a sensor of its own; it is attuned to the wavelengths and frequencies most similar to the neurons between it.

The pressure, capacitance, and ability of the node to change and interchange voltages at its sites are pre-described by its neuron on either end. There are many other sophisticated, powerful connections between the nodes able to dictate the exact mechanisms, methodologies, polices, and programs that are used in the transmissions of messages between cells. This communication is one of the most important functions of a cell body; therefore the emissaries to be entrusted with the messages are selected for their ability to reproduce.

Nucleus of the Schwann Cell

The nucleus of the Schwann cell is a directive mechanism, which is part of the neurilemma. As was described in other paragraphs, the neurilemma (an ectodermic structure) is a skin with an extremely sensitive characteristic from which skin structures, nervous systems, and special senses and activities develop. These are usually endocrine in nature, especially those that are coordinative with the anterior pituitary and the adrenal glands. Since the neurilemma is composed of Schwann cells, it is able to encircle the myelin sheath, protecting the axon. The neurilemma is a highly protective and sensitive device; the nucleated Schwann cells there help the myelin sheath increase the conduction rate of axon transmissions.

One specific capability of the Schwann cell's nucleus is to coordinate and direct hydrolyzation, the movement of water (H_2O) around the cell membrane, to coordinate the conduction of highly charged atomic particles through the axon.

While examining nervous and muscular tissues under a microscope, physiologist Theodor Schwann discovered the cells that envelope nerve fibers—the Schwann cells.

He also discovered the digestive enzyme he named pepsin (Greek pepsis, meaning to digest) but when he claimed that yeast was alive, he was ridiculed by his peers for subscribing to vitalism.

His famous quote "all living things are composed of cells and cell products" led to the cell theory and became the foundation for modern histology.

www.LifeEnergyResearch.com

The nucleus of the Schwann cell directs and dictates placement of cells. The neurilemma and the myelin sheath dictate to reject any materials not belonging in the system. This is a demarcation process, which cordons off areas of operation to the axon.

A highly specific screening process can be coordinated with the nucleus of the Schwann cell. The integrity and the insistence of purity around the system are indicative of the clean operation of axon transmissions.

The vaporization of super-charged gas particles act in harmonic laser-fashion between the exchanges of neurons (cell bodies and central processes) and can be coordinated and controlled by the nucleus of the Schwann cell. These nuclei hold a great deal of power, for if they were to fail, the signals coming from cell bodies that need to be received by other neurons would disperse. Therefore, there would be an erratic pattern, with the goals, dreams, and desires of the organism and the individual being shattered.

The conditions of nervousness that occur in human beings are frequently related to a buildup of highly charged particles that are not being readily processed from one axon to the next. The cause for nervousness can be manifold, however, in certain situations, the nucleus of the Schwann cell can help to coordinate the movement of energy in a harmonic way so as to avoid any emotional disturbances.

The location and quality of operation is often dictated by the nucleus of the Schwann cell, due to the fact that it has the ability to coordinate the protective membranes holding the myelin sheath and the axon in place.

Chapter Four

> *The conditions of nervousness that occur in human beings are frequently related to a buildup of highly charged particles that are not being readily processed from one axon to the next.*
>
> *The cause for nervousness can have an assortment of features, however, the nucleus of the Schwann cell can help to coordinate the movement of energy in a harmonic way so as to avoid any emotional disturbances.*

The equalization processes of the peripheral activities of the body are evaluated and coordinated by the nucleus of the Schwann cell. This nucleus contains abilities that are similar to endocrine structures. It can operate automatically under the directive of the governor mechanisms and be tuned to grant many specific operational powers to these cells.

Chapter 4.—Advanced SAF® View

The organs and glands primarily affected are: lungs (7), skin (19), thymus immune (1), bones and muscles (9), kidneys (16), adrenals (13), pancreas (20, and parathyroid (22).

Neuroglial Cells (Glial or Glia)

"*Neuro*" means nervous system and "*glial*" translates as glue. This was long thought to be the glue of the nervous system, and although that view has changed, the neuroglial cells are the greatest in number and are part of the supporting element of the central nervous system (CNS) and the peripheral nervous system (PNS). These special cells insulate one neuron from another, destroy and remove pathogens, provide homeostasis, form the myelin, and provide nutrients and oxygen to neurons. The neuroglial surrounds the axon and allows the axon to transmit its encoded messages without disturbance from the outside, and without the dispersion of energy from the inside. This encapsulated area prevents any interference from altering the message in transit from one neuron to the next.

In the PNS, the glial cells are the Schwann cells.

Preventing the system from being overrun by infection or interference from the outside is an ability of the neuroglial cell. It can also transmutate its configuration to protect the axon from different environmental interferences. This is due to the fact that the axon is constantly changing its transmission modes from stepping up or stepping down voltages, to modulating frequencies and wavelengths.

Neuroglial cells hold onto or contain actions of the axon, which may be toxic to it. The residues of highly charged atomic particles are extremely small and unseen, even on microscopic scales, and are part of a specific waste disposal that is part of the neuroglial activity. This detoxification process is extremely necessary so that the transmission of energies from one nerve cell to the other can proceed without interference from errant internal structures.

The neuroglial cells making up the myelin sheath act as a protective mechanism, preventing any adverse energies from entering while permitting the axon to communicate freely with its neighbors.

The recording mechanism of the neuroglial cell is like that of the dendrite and the axon in its ability to observe and record incidents and energies as they pass through. These inscriptions are deeply set into the neuroglial cell and can be retrieved from any point in time. The compression of energy taking place within the neuroglial cell lets it record up to and beyond 1,000 years, so the system has been set up to allow a constant, almost immortal survival.

The methodologies of operation concerning the neuroglial cell are the coordination and communication of encoded messages proceeding from one axon to the next in the form of prismatic, highly charged atomic particles. These geometrically shaped atomic particles can be transmitted and exchanged by vaporization, which is a transportational mechanism causing energy to appear and disappear in one place and then appear and disappear in the next place. This activity is part of a communication process similar to that used by a telephone company or the world wide web.

Finally, the neuroglial cell has the ability to hold motion and coordinate activity around itself. It has the sense and intelligence that is inferior only to that of the nucleus of the Schwann cell and the central control processes of the neuron itself.

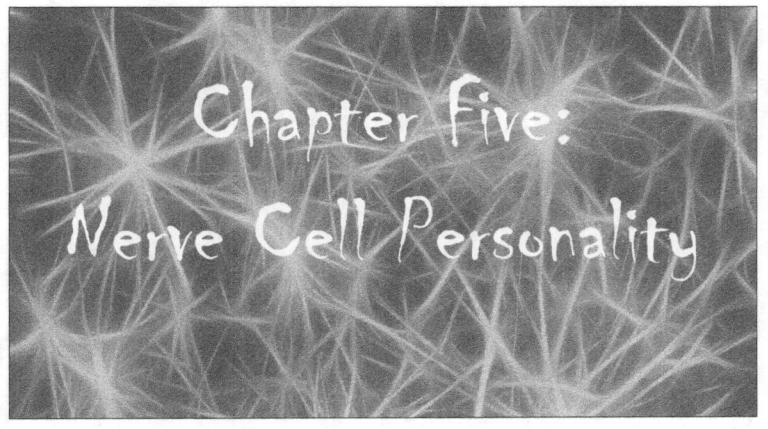

Chapter Five: Nerve Cell Personality

> *"Like Proteus, the first god who was able to perfect transmutation, the ions are able to change into any shape whatsoever."*
>
> —Joseph R. Scogna, Jr

Neurons are classified by the number of processes or poles associated with each cell body.

- ***Unipolar**—one process extends from the cell body. Simple messages of light, sound, and temperature.*

- ***Bipolar**—two poles emerge at either end or from the same point. These are considered the specialized sensory neurons for the transmission of the sense of smell, sight, taste, hearing and balance.*

- ***Multipolar**—a single long axon, many dendrite branches to be able to take in much information from other neurons. This is the most intelligent and largest neural group in the body.*

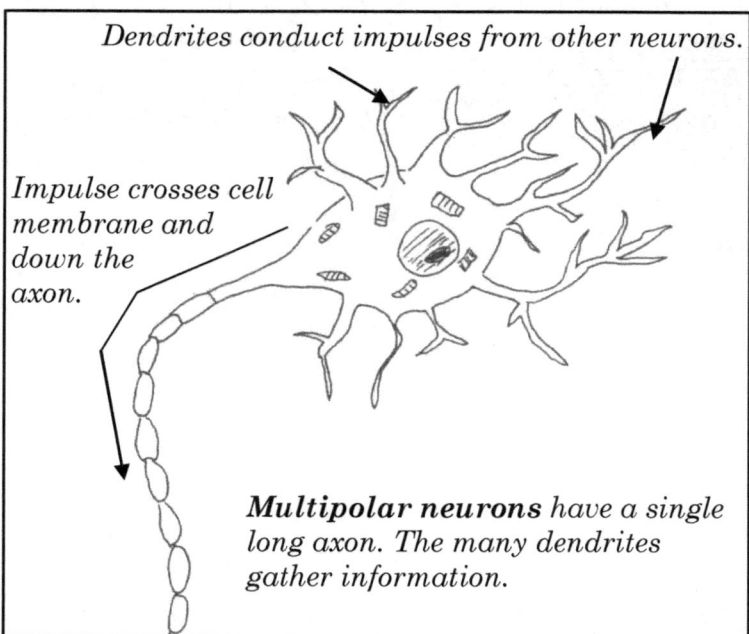

Dendrites conduct impulses from other neurons.

Impulse crosses cell membrane and down the axon.

***Multipolar neurons** have a single long axon. The many dendrites gather information.*

Ions

The ion was named by Michael Faraday, using the Greek word for "going". He had found "something moving" through a solution from one electrode to another and called it an ion.

Ions are highly charged atomic particles or agitated atoms. It is highly charged because the number of electrons is not equal to the number of protons. When an atom loses one or more electrons it has a positive charge; if it gains an electron it holds a negative charge.

An atom is agitated with the intent and necessity of sending a message. The modulation or shaking of specific atoms will create a certain configuration, pattern, or "picture" which can be broadcast through the neural system. When these atoms are moved through the system from one neural cell to the next, moving rapidly across each nerve cell membrane in turn, this picture of a survival plan to increase the harmony in the system can be relayed from one location to the next. It is much like advertising on television.

When immediately set into an organized harmonic agitation pattern, the ions are able to selectively accept or filter poisons from their systems. This means that once a message is put or encoded on atomic structures, it prevents any other message from interfering with it. It is broadcast with the intent of being heard.

Because they are transmutational, once the ions are encoded with a message and the message is received, a neuron may take the very same atoms and re-agitate them into a different specific pattern, without loss of energy. This process is a very specialized part of fusion energy (creation of energy from nothing), which has been borrowed from the mind and the spirit.

The ions can be digested, absorbed, reabsorbed, and dissolved. They can change configuration, move back and forth and change into many different shapes. Like Proteus, the first god who was able to perfect transmutation, the ions are able to change into any shape whatsoever. They work in much the same manner as a television transmission changes from one program or channel to the next.

It is glorious to know that these energies can be rearranged and broadcast into any pattern that one wishes. In this sense, an individual can be infinitely happy and never worry about loss of energy from one activity to the next (if he can master light and dark pressures).

Accepting their directives well, the ions mold themselves into entities. However, it is the neurons, the DNA and RNA, and all the governing structures of the body that set the ions into motion patterns of harmony. This harmonic pattern is the one most sought after for the genetic plan of the body and has long since been able to analyze the overall structure and configuration of this universe. Since this is a universe of harmony, disharmony dismantles it.

On a harmonic wavelength and frequency, an individual can survive for extreme lengths of time. In disharmonic states, the body dissolves very rapidly. Disharmonic states simply do not belong in this universe. They are pushed outside to universes of disharmony. Therefore, it is extremely important that we exercise the potential of harmony and organization in

> *On a harmonic wavelength and frequency, an individual can survive for extreme lengths of time. In disharmonic states, the body dissolves very rapidly. Disharmonic states simply do not belong in this universe.*

the body demonstrated by the neurons and the governor mechanisms of the body.

Once programmed, the ions are sent into a configuration of energy helping to establish the quality and location of the message itself. The ions are a statement of the neuron and of the DNA. It is almost as if one were to say that a greeting card from a certain family member is a statement of how much they care about the receiver. Anything sent from a specific location qualifies that site. If a nasty letter is sent from a particular place, then that area has been qualified as a source of disharmony. If a loving, very interesting and provocative letter is sent from a locality, then that letter will qualify that spot as interesting and harmonic. It is the same with ions; they qualify the sender.

The message of the ion is often one of attraction and similarity. They teach lessons of coordinating harmonies in the body, reproducing oneself, and changing into different structures using the same basic energies. It is the reproductive method and the action of coordinating harmonies from one step to the next that produces a state of chronic existence, or immortality.

Unipolar Neuron

The unipolar neuron is a simple nerve cell with only one process or pole. It has one specific message: to increase harmony and the overall survival potential.

The ability of the mechanism to reproduce itself is part of the survival message that is encoded or inscripted upon the unipolar neuron. This information being sent to other neurons is reproduced so it may grow and prosper. The idea is that an individual is only as happy and harmonic as he is productive. This is a very special and important message, one that is broadcast through the idea of constant creation, since this is a universe of creative ability and harmonic energies. Thus, harmonic creation is the message of the unipolar neuron.

However, exchangeability of the unipolar neuron's message is creativity in a very light sense. The message does not say to create masses, but to create energies of thought and of vapor, ethereal energies inducing large masses to automatically create. A writer may compose a poem and 150 years later, have a structure erected in his name; this exemplifies the idea that thought can coerce mass into specific shapes and forms.

The coordination of activities in the system specifically dictates that there be some directive forces coming from the single-minded unipolar neuron. Its

This is a universe of creative ability and harmonic energies. An individual is only as happy and harmonic as he is productive.

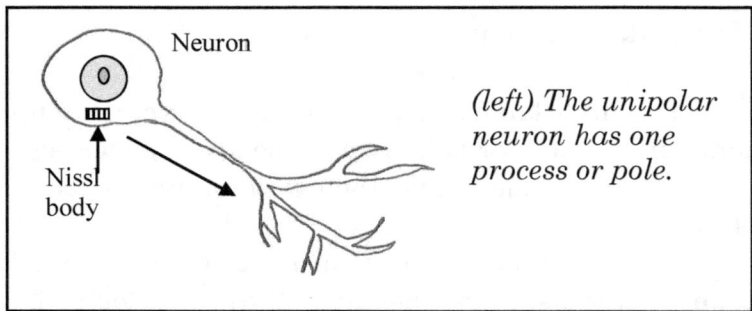

(left) The unipolar neuron has one process or pole.

directives are straightforward and to the point; it says, "Create."

The digestive dissolution capabilities of the neuron are practiced. It is constantly observing new ways and better conditions for reproduction. Its main bent is survival. Therefore, it is continually observing and digesting information from other neurons which may coerce it to change its mind from being unipolar to being bipolar or multipolar in function. If this neuron decides to do this, it may take its cylindrical chromophils or Nissl bodies and convert them into axon hillocks. These axon hillocks would then reach out, providing an axon structure and highly coordinated multi-faceted purposes for the neuron instead of a unipolar activity.

Another function of the unipolar neuron is to detoxify and contain the system, preventing it from losing sight of the one purpose of creation.

The unipolar neuron directly coordinates much of the running and synchronization of electrostatic and electrodynamic energy in the system. It is able to coordinate and consent to the relegation of highly charged atoms from one neuron to the next, creating patterns of harmony in the body.

Bipolar Neuron

The bipolar neuron has two processes or poles with which to handle impulses. These two poles move out from the neuron and allow a push-pull of energy. This may be the basic electrical function of all history, in that the individual has moved from direct current in the unipolar cell to direct alternating current in a bipolar function. The bipolar neuron is much more coordinated than the unipolar neuron, which only sees one creative force; it can see neither black nor white, dark nor light, just its own specific energy. The bipolar is able to understand both the positives and negatives.

The nerve tracks of the bipolar neuron are interesting in that they have the capability to reject ideas. This means that the bipolar neuron does not need to broadcast the same pattern and the same message all the time. It is mainly interested in broadcasting an idea it deems necessary for a better quality harmony. Thus, the second function of the bipolar neuron is to assess quality. It is interested in a more precise type of intelligence, rather than just continual existence. It is survival with great dignity that is desired here.

In this way, the bipolar neuron filters out information that is not compatible with its overall purposes.

The bipolar neuron is much more coordinated than the unipolar neuron, because it can see creative force and different energies. It can see black and white, dark and light; it is able to understand both the positives and negatives.

www.LifeEnergyResearch.com

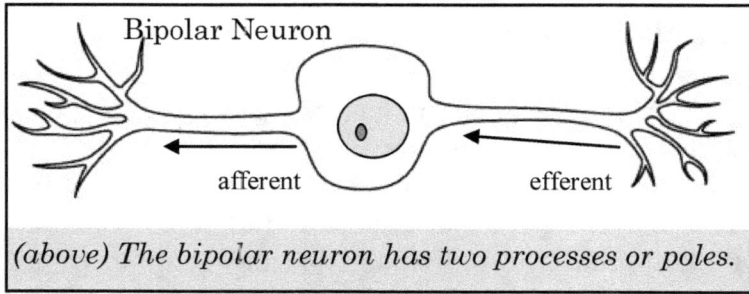

(above) The bipolar neuron has two processes or poles.

The circulation of ideas in the system is extremely important to the overall process of the bipolar neuron. It is disseminating these concepts to other nerve cells, trying to upgrade the entire information broadcasting system necessary for one to exist with the ability to discern right from wrong and light from dark. A straightforward, continual creation that demands production without being sensible cannot be the only activity of the overall mechanism. The case for the system, however, really depends upon the ability of cells to mature. As neurons direct various nerve functions in the body, the communication between cellular bodies and tissues in the entire organization begin to side with neurons that have the most potential force. The neurons that can control power in the system are going to be the ones that are listened to most. Many of the corrective measures that are taken within the system are not necessarily connected to a system-wide unbridled attempt at survival, but a more selective, quality existence.

The bipolar neuron also has the ability to augment itself. The dissemination of its ideas is extremely important to the coordination and communication of other neurons and cellular bodies within the entire organism. The bipolar neuron is an individual nerve cell that likes to campaign and win other cells over to its side.

Extremely important to the complete running of the system, the bipolar neuron is different from the unipolar neuron in that it does not have a one-value logic for creation. It has a two-value logic, considering the idea of creation and destruction, as well. It chooses things to create and not to create and is selective about its production.

Pseudounipolar Neuron

A sub-type of bipolar neuron is the pseudounipolar neuron, with one axon and two split branches (not dendrites); one branch goes to the central nervous system (CNS), the other to the peripheral nervous system (PNS).

This may be a unipolar neuron in the process of becoming a bipolar neuron, or a bipolar neuron downgrading to a unipolar neuron.

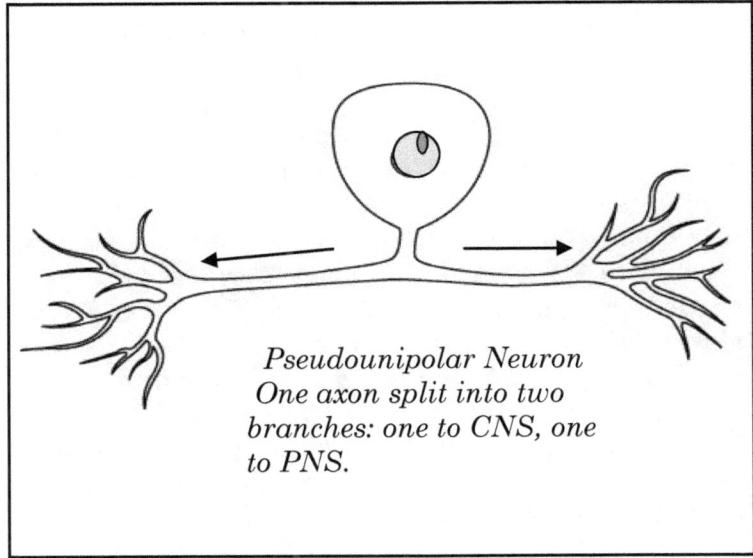

Pseudounipolar Neuron
One axon split into two branches: one to CNS, one to PNS.

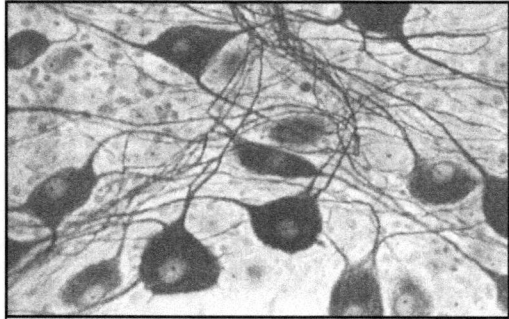

(left) Vagus nerves are one of 12 pairs of cranial nerves that branch through the body. Vagus (Latin) means "wandering."

Electric Shock Then and Now

The bipolar vagus nerve is both an afferent sensory and an efferent motor nerve with portals in the brain stem. It is implicated in several syndromes, including bipolar depression and epilepsy.

Triggers for bipolar depression can be a traumatic life event, drug use (narcotic, recreational, thyroid and prednisone), appetite suppressants, cold remedies, and even excessive caffeine intake.

Anti-depressant drugs often set off episodes of mania requiring additional drugs.

In cases of epilepsy, triggers can be a brain injury or tumor, drug and alcohol misuse, toxin ingestion or infections of the central nervous system from bacterium, virus, fungus, amoeba or algae.

When drugs to do not quell the syndromes (called "treatment-resistant or drug-resistant") vagus nerve stimulation (VNS) is sometimes employed, in which a pacemaker-type device is surgically implanted in the chest with wires and electrodes that stimulate the vagus nerves in the neck. It is the terrifying electric shock of the past now in a new guise.

It is hoped that increased knowledge and awareness of the inner workings of our holistic system will change the direction of humankind regarding any disorders and dysfunctions, and propel us instead in the direction of harmony and balance.

Chapter Five

Multipolar Neuron

By definition, the multipolar neuron can have as many processes as necessary, at least more than two. The many branch-like processes, called dendrites, conduct impulses to the neural cell body from many different neurons.

It first appears that the multipolar neuron is more astute when it comes to intelligence and imagination. However, it sacrifices the ability of base line survival for the concoction of a very special communication process. It is the "Einstein cell." These are the cells that are found in the medulla oblongata and the pons. These sophisticated cells, named Purkinje, like to consider from an omni-viewpoint. They enjoy observing the conditions and things removed from "to be or not to be" and escalated to the idea of "maybe." This cell considers the finer details of existence.

The multipolar neuron has the ability to partake of much of the activity going on around it. It likes to spend time looking at energies and dissecting them.

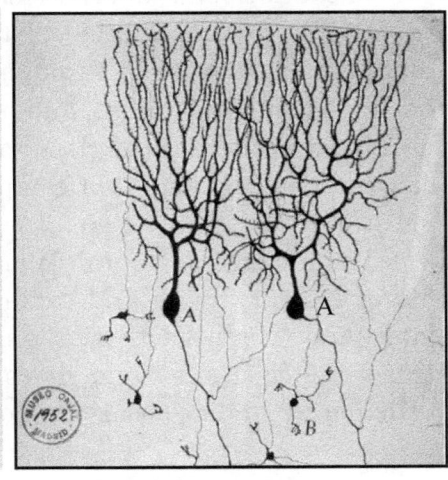

(right) An 1899 drawing of pigeon nerve cells, A, a Purkinje neuron, with its arbor of dendrites.
Purkinje was named for a Czech anatomist, Jan Evangelista Purknye.

www.LifeEnergyResearch.com

> *The multipolar neuron is greatly enthused about the idea of creating a higher quality mechanism. The information is monitored by the DNA and RNA molecule. The energies moving into the cellular structure of the multipolar neuron will create cell-splitting activities in the organism, which may eventually, in years to come, produce a superhuman being.*

It is eclectic, but not to a fault, choosing to use many axioms of nature, which can be coordinated into a complex principle of survival.

The multipolar neuron is often capable of decontaminating highly charged, excited atoms, which may or may not be rejected by the simpler neurons. This multipolar neuron spends a good deal of time observing the characteristics of the messages that are sent to it by other neurons. The multipolar neuron spends much of its time considering a very artistic communication to send to other neurons, while the unipolar and bipolar neurons are sending repetitious and highly unimaginative messages.

The multipolar neuron, for the sake of its own protection, frequently rejects the superfluous information being broadcast throughout the system. It sits back in its inner chamber and observes and thinks on its own primitive level. It is a highly sophisticated computer mechanism, but compared to the mind and spirit has a long way to go.

The multipolar neuron is probably the most capable of memory trace and experience recall. It calculates and weighs activities and energies that have transpired in the system. It counts wins and losses, utilizing its ability observing possibilities for the best attack profile to use against viruses, toxins, pests, chemicals, errant frequencies and other types of invader forces in the body that inhibit the gross survival operations of the organism.

The multipolar neuron is greatly enthused about the idea of creating a higher quality mechanism. In many ways, the information that is fed back from the multipolar neuron is monitored by the DNA and RNA molecule. The energies moving into the cellular structure of the multipolar neuron will create cell-splitting activities in the organism, which may eventually, in years to come, produce a superhuman being.

Finally, the multipolar neuron spends much time protecting itself and its ideas. It has a capability of disturbing the delicate structure of memory and coordination with the cell, sensing energy in the environment that is highly agitated in nature, especially electrons, gamma particles, and x-rays. One of the premiere protective directives of the multipolar neuron is the directive to avoid losing any of its peripheral processes, for it is these that allow it to be a multipolar. With the destruction of peripheral processes, the multipolar neuron may backslide into a bipolar or even a unipolar activity.

Chapter 5.—Advanced SAF® View

The organs and glands primarily affected are: digestion (4), sex organs (8), pancreas (20), heart (2), colon (3), kidneys (16), spleen (23).

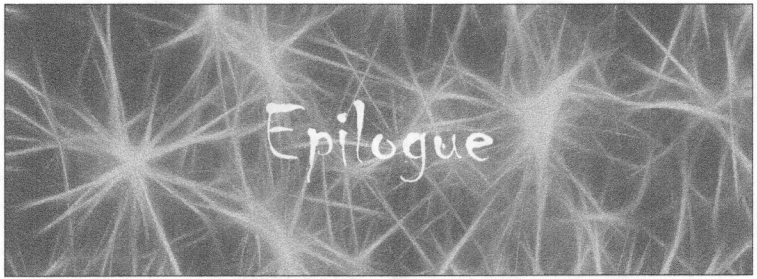

Epilogue

In going through the files after Joe's death, I came upon a simple 1984 manuscript. Notations indicated it coordinated with an SAF® computer program for the Apple IIe, entitled Neuron/Axon (110-23 6R), Grade 1.250, which was also located in the files.

This special book gives the reader another dimension for understanding the universe by examining its most subtle energy level, noted in the SAF® lineup as #12, the brain and nervous system.

Joseph Scogna understood well that subtle energy could have more impact on a human than a gross form of energy. Whatever occurs or causes an effect on a cellular or quantum level will cause an effect simultaneously on the greater level of organized Life Energy, a human being, with ramifications for family, community, animals, and even projects out to the greater cosmos.

In *Light, Dark*, Joe examines the invisible areas of the human being. We live in a harmonic universe—it was not created out of chaos. Scogna explains that the actions of the individual cells are geared toward survival and reproduce themselves following that genetic, harmonic plan.

Just before writing this book, Joe had completed much of his work with frequency counters and infrared detectors to locate what he called the gravinomet-

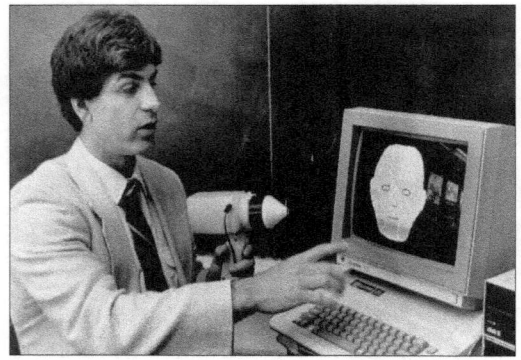

Joseph R. Scogna, Jr. explaining his computing system, with infrared "gun" in hand. 1986.

ric or nervous system "venting sites" on the body. At these spots, the nerves relating to specific organs and glands release their invisible, heated energy. By his own calculation, there are thousands of such sites on the human body.

Joe cataloged and digitized trends and syndromes on how the energies of the body interact and what the various combinations of symptoms meant.

"Pain," he said, "is simply the body trying to speak, trying to communicate a source of trouble."

Because the body doesn't speak English or any language as we know it, we have to get it to speak to us on its terms, which is pressure and space, pain and sensation. Our symptoms, then, our sensations, aches, pains, and emotions are messages we were meant to decode. The language for decoding these is both a mathematical and a grammatical language called SAF® (Self Awareness Formulas), which uses a combination of numbers and words to depict our physical and mental aspects, emotions, and attitudes, along with 128 sensory channels. It is an ancient-future speak already built into the DNA of humankind, and one we can readily learn.

The reader will note a few of the organ and gland

Kathy M. Scogna at an SAF® workshop, 2013

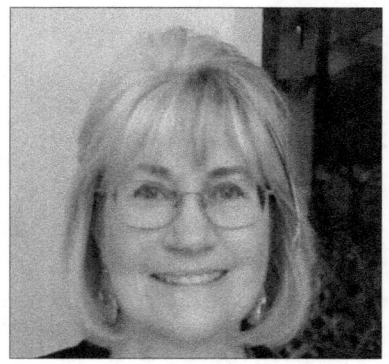

systems affected at the end of each chapter, as Advanced SAF® work. With a practitioner's help, the reader can access the SAFonline database for what pertains to a personal SAF® chain sequence.

The theory and numbering system of the SAF® language is found in *SAF Simplified*. The background information can be located in *The Promethion: A Comprehensive Study of the Principles of Life Energy,* and especially in *Junk DNA: Unlocking the Hidden Secrets of Your DNA*. The hardwiring of the universe plus the activities of the Genetic Planning Mechanism (GPM) with the 128 sense perceptions of humankind are all ensconced in our DNA.

In *Light, Dark,* Joe writes of the neuron, axon, Schwann cell, myelin sheath and other aspects of the nervous system as if these are alive, endowed with personality, intentions, dreams and desires... and so they are!

Our comprehension of the subtle, invisible communication links within us allows for the greater holographic image of the human to be revealed.

—Kathy M. Scogna

www.LifeEnergyResearch.com

Acknowledgments

Special thanks to Kalli Marie Scogna for her diligent hours at the keyboard one summer long ago, so that this volume could be taken out of the darkness of the files and into the light of day.

Thanks to Nic Scogna for capturing the dendrite image used on the front cover and chapter headings.

References and Further Reading

The Anatomy Coloring Book, Winn Kapit and Lawrence M. Elson (1977).
Dictionary of Science, Webster's New World, Helicon Publishing Ltd, 1998
The Human Body series, The Nervous System: Circuits of Communication, Torstar Books (1985).
Light, Dark (manuscript), Joseph R. Scogna, Jr., 1984
Neurons-Axons, SAF® computer program, 1983
Wikipedia

Other Scogna Books:
- Amino Acids: A Nutritional Guide
- Dialogue with Joseph R. Scogna, Jr.
- Homeopathy Revisited: A Modern Energetic View of an Ancient Healing Art
- Interview with Joe Scogna, 1982
- Junk DNA: Unlocking the Hidden Secrets of Your DNA
- Nutrionics
- The Promethion: A Comprehensive Study of the Principles of Life Energy
- The SAF® Infrared Manual
- SAF® Modality Sorter
- SAF® Road Map, Level 1 Training
- SAF® Simplified
- SAF® Training Manual, Level 2
- The Secret of SAF®
- The Threat of the Poison Reign: A Treatise on Electromagnetic Pollution
- Project Isis: The Fundamentals of Human Electricity
- What Your Blood Tells You: Energetic, Nutritional Answers for Change

www.LifeEnergyResearch.com

Credits

front cover: (ignited dendrites), PixBay

p 7 (vagus nerve cells) Biophoto Associates (1985)
p 12 (nerve cell) illustration by Kathy M. Scogna, Scogna Library
p 28 (DNA). Scogna Library
p 34 (neurons and nerve endings) (adapted) illustration by Winn Kapit (1977)
p 42 (dendrite) illustration by Kathy M. Scogna
p 50 (protection of the system- myelin and neurilemma) adapted illustration by Kathy M. Scogna
p 66 (multipolar neuron) illustration by Kathy M. Scogna
p 72 (unipolar neuron) Wikipedia
p 74 (bipolar neuron) Wikipedia
p 75 (pseudounipolar neuron), Wikipedia
p 76 (vagus nerve cells) Biophoto Associates (1985)
p 77 (Purkinje cell) drawing by Santiago Ramon y Cajal (1899), Wikipedia
p 82 (photo of Joseph R. Scogna, Jr) Reading-Eagle Times newspaper(1986), Scogna Library
p 83 (photo of Kathy M. Scogna) by Myrna Hallett (2013) Scogna Library

back cover (nerve cell) illustration by Kathy M. Scogna

www.LifeEnergyResearch.com

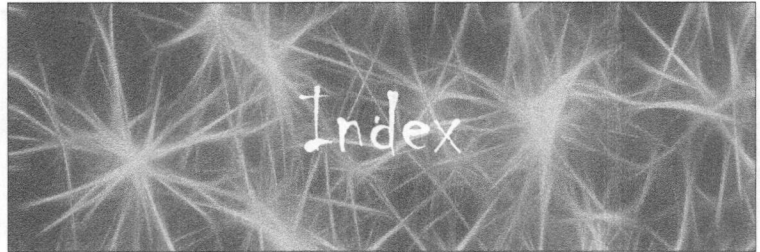

Index

A
Action potential, 51
Adrenal glands, 26, 59, 65
Afferent, 35, 39, 74, 76
Agitated atom, 67
Amperes, 26
Analyzation, 15, 29, 46
Ancient-future speak, 82
Anterior pituitary, 59
Anti-depressants, 76
Autoimmune, 54
Axon hillock, 12, 25-26, 72
Axon, 45-47

B
Balance, 66, 76
Bipolar (ill.), 74
Bipolar depression, 76
Bipolar neuron, 73
Blueprint, 17, 29
Body is a hologram, 33
Bones and Muscles, 19, 20, 62
Brain, 23, 26, 53, 81

C
Central process, 38, 37-39
Chapter 1. SAF View, 26
Chapter 2. SAF View, 32
Chapter 3. SAF view, 47
Chapter 4. SAF View, 62
Chapter 5. SAF View, 79
Chapter Five: nerve cell personality, 65
Chapter Four: protection of the system, 49
Chapter One: the nerve cell, 11
Chapter Three: operations, 33
Chapter Two: command center, 27
Chromophil, 23-24
Colon, 26, 79
Color, love for, 23, 24
Command center, 27
Computer chip, 13
Computer, 9, 13, 78, 81
Controls life energy, 14,
Create, 72
Creation (s), 7,13,19,20,31,68, 71,72,74,75
Cytoplasm, 19-20

D
Decoding language, 82
Depression, 76
Dendrite (ill.), 42
Dendrites, 41-43
Detoxification, 19, 25, 30, 63
Demarcating/tion, 53, 55, 60
Demyelinating disease, 54
Digestion, 19, 41, 57, 79
Disharmonic states, 69
Disharmony, 51, 52, 68, 69
DNA (ill.), 28
DNA, 13, 28, 29, 30, 31, 68, 69, 78, 79, 82, 83, 84
DNA, language is in the, 82

www.LifeEnergyResearch.com

Index

E
Eastern philosophies, 8
Ectodermic, 59
Efferent, 35, 39, 74, 76
Einstein cell, 77
Electric charge, 49, 51, 53, 54
Electric forces, 15
Electric pressure, 13, 18, 39, 43, 54
Electric shock, 76
Electrochemical 14, 17, 19, 29, 55
Electromagnetic, 15, 18, 23, 26
Endocrine system, 26, 47, 59, 61
Endoplasmic, 21
Endowed with personality, 83
Environment/al, 17, 18, 20, 29, 30, 41, 45, 63, 79
Enzymes, 21, 22
Epilepsy, 76
Epilogue, 81
Evaluation, 17, 29, 51
ExTech IR 200, 90

F
Faraday, Michael, 67
Fire, 51, 52
Framework of energy, 13
Frequency (ies) 17, 35, 38, 68, 69, 79, 81
Functions of neurons and nerve endings (ill), 34, 35

G
Galaxies in night sky, 7
Genesis, 7
Genetic structure, 13
Genetic, 9, 13, 14, 17, 29, 31, 38, 68, 81, 83, 90
Glial (glia), 63-65
Glue of the system, 63
Grammatical language, 82, 91
Gravinometric venting sites, 81-82

H
Harmonic universe, 81
Harmonic wavelengths, 69
Harmony, 51, 52, 67, 68, 69, 71, 72, 73, 76
Heart, 47, 79
Hologram/holograph, 33, 38, 39, 83
Holographic view of body, 39
Homeostasis, 29, 38, 63
Huygens, Christian 8
Hydrolyzation, 59
Hypothalamus, 23, 32

I
Impulse, 22, 51-52
Infrared detectors, 81, 90
Infrared, 9, 38, 39, 52, 81, 90, 91
Introduction, 7
Ions, 67-69

J
Junk DNA, 13, 30, 83, 90

K
Kidneys, 62, 79

L
Language is in the DNA, 82
Let there be light, 7
Life energy, 8, 9, 14, 31, 80
Light and dark, 9, 11, 13, 17, 22, 25, 35, 37, 38, 68
Light and electricity, 7
Light is a corpuscle, 8
Light is wave motion, 7
Liver, 26
Love for color, 23, 24
Lungs, 62
Lysosomes, 21, 22

Light, Dark

M
Memory, 9, 55, 78, 79
Mental, 28, 32, 82
Mind, 18, 26, 68, 72, 78
Mirrored blueprint, 29
Multiple sclerosis, 54
Multipolar neuron (ill.), 66
Multipolar neuron, 77-79
Myelin sheath and neurilemma (ill.), 50
Myelin sheath, 53-54

N
Nerve cell (ill.), 12
Nerve cell personality, 65
Nerve cell, 11, 13-14
Nervous system = #12, 9, 81
Nervousness, 61
Neurilemma, 55
Neuroglial, 63-65
Neuron/switch mechanism, 11, 13
Neuron, 13-14
Neuron, nerve cell (ill.), 12
Neurons classified, 66
Neurosecretory, 23
Newton, Sir, Isaac, 8
Nissl Bodies, 12, 21-22, 23, 25, 72
Node of Ranvier, 57-58
Nuclear magnetic resonance, 17, 18
Nucleolus, 17-18
Nucleus of the neuron, 13, 15
Nucleus of the Schwann cell, 59-61

O
Ohms, 19, 25, 26, 51
Old Testament, 7
Operations, 33
Organic functions, 8
Organs and glands, 9, 27, 32, 47, 62, 79, 82, 91

P
Pain and sensation, 82
Pain is the body trying to speak, 82
Pancreas, 23, 62, 79
Parathyroid, 23, 47, 62
Particle and a wave, 8
Perception of time, 43
Peripheral and Central Process, 38
Peripheral process, 35-36
Personality, 9, 65-79, 82
Pigeon nerve cell, 77
Pituitary, 23, 26, 59
Planck, Max, 8
Potassium, 51
Pressure and space, 13, 15, 36, 82
Pressures (light), 15
Protection of the system, 49
Protein, 19, 20, 21, 22, 23, 31, 37
Proteus, 65, 68
Pseudounipolar (ill.), 75
Pseudounipolar, 75
Purkinje, 77
Purkinje nerve cell (ill.), 77
Pyramidal structure, 23

Q
Quantum theory/mechanics, 8
Quantum, 8, 81

R
Radiant, 8
Radio, 17, 21, 38
Record experiences, 42, 55
Recording/record, 42, 43, 46, 55, 64
Records information, 46
RNA, 27, 29, 30, 31-32, 68, 78, 79
Repair, mending, 53, 54

Index

S
SAF® #12, 9, 81
SAF® Infrared Manual, 91
SAF® language, 9, 82
SAF® number sequences, 9
SAF Simplified, 83, 91
SAF® 9, 26, 28, 32, 38, 47, 62, 79, 81, 82, 83, 91
Schwann, Theodor, 59
Scogna, Joseph R, 9, 11, 27, 33, 49, 65, 81-83
Scogna, Kalli Marie, 84
Scogna, Kathy M., *photo*, 83
Scogna, Nic, 84
Self Awareness Formulas, 82
Sex organs, 79
Skin, 47, 59, 62
Sodium, 51
Space/spaces, 13, 15, 18, 29, 36, 46, 57, 82
Spaces (dark), 15
Spirit/spiritual, 18, 28, 32, 68, 78
Spleen, 32, 79
Stimulation of vagus nerve, 76
Superhuman being, 79
Switch mechanism (light/dark), 11, 13

T
Teleportation, 57
Tempo, 13, 18, 26, 27, 31
Thymus-immune, 62
Thyroid, 23, 26, 47, 62
Time and space, 36, 46
Time passes slowly/quickly, 42-43
Timing mechanism, 15, 18
Transfer of energy, 8
Transmissions, 35, 46, 55, 58, 59, 60
Transmitter, 21
Transmutation, 21, 25, 37, 53, 65, 67, 68

U
Ultrasonic, 17
Unipolar (ill.), 72
Unipolar neuron, 71
Universe of creative ability, 71

V
VNS, 76
Vagus nerve, 76
Vaporization, 53, 57, 60, 64,
Veins and arteries, 47
Venting sites, nerves, 9, 82
Voltage, 38, 39, 43, 45, 58, 63

W
What our symptoms mean, 8, 91

Where to get Books and IR Device mentioned

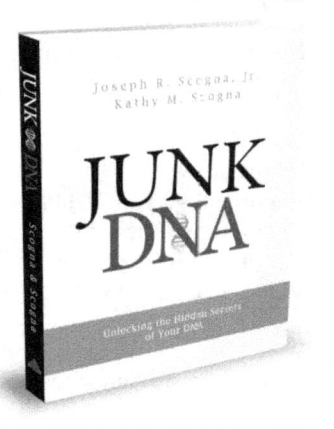

Junk DNA: Unlocking the Hidden Secrets of Your DNA

98% of DNA material has been declared "genetic gibberish, junk"?

We know better!

Open the pages of this book and unlock the secrets in that hidden 98%.

- *Superman Seminar with ROM and RAM in our DNA*
- *The Story of Z (the unknowns, alchemy, the elements)*
- *16 Steps of the Z Process*
- *128 Sensory Channels, detailed descriptions*
- *The Allergy Connection, with fascinating case histories and explanations!*

A serious study, but reader-friendly

Purchase at Amazon.com & CreateSpace.com

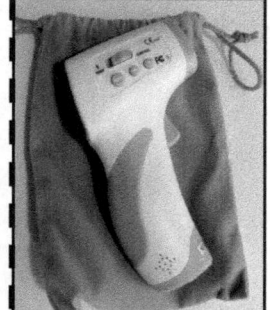

ExTech IR 200 is the Infrared device to use to create an SAF® chain of numbers. Inexpensive, easy to use!

Complete instructions in *The SAF Infrared Manual* (next page)

ExTech IR 200
Purchase at Amazon.com

www.LifeEnergyResearch.com

SAF® is truly the Rosetta Stone for the body, mind & spirit!

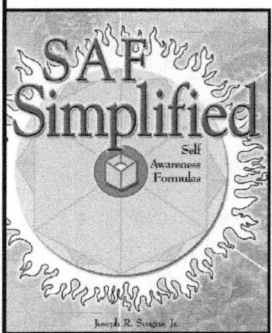

Our symptoms are messages we were meant to decode! The language for decoding is both a mathematical and a grammatical language, a combination of numbers and words to depict organs & glands, emotions, attitudes, and functions across many subjects.

The theory, the numbering system, the organs and glands, the emotions, and the basics of how to read a chain sequence.

Purchase *SAF Simplified* at www.LifeEnergyResearch.com

Purchase *The SAF Infrared Manual* at Amazon.com or CreateSpace.com

Purchase the IR 200 at Amazon.com

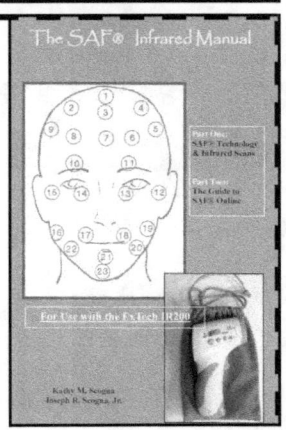

- Learn about Infrared use in SAF® work. Read fascinating **stories and case studies**. Temperature template to follow.
- How to Use the SAFonline service (free for students, small fee for practitioners—by day, week, month, yr).
- **Step by Step: How to use the IR200 Infrared device** and Questionnaires with SAFonline.
- Based on chain sequence, **how to find Remedies** and Interpretations; details of the 40 categories, how to use these.

www.LifeEnergyResearch.com

www.ingramcontent.com/pod-product-compliance
Lightning Source LLC
Chambersburg PA
CBHW071748170526
45167CB00003B/982